The Resting Body Diet: The Quick Easy Guide to the Metabolic weight loss diet

by T. Flora

ISBN-13:
978-1974533916

ISBN-10:
1974533913

Table of Contents

1. Introduction

I want to thank you for your interest in this book.

I conducted a lot of research and compacted just the highlighted notes on the metabolic diet as a beginner's quick reference guide. I hope that you like it and that it can help you look and feel better.

2. Chapter 1: What is HEC? (Hellish hormones, Energy, Calories)

Hormones control metabolism, not Calories. Hormones determine what type of weight you will lose and where you may lose it from but not the Calories. Hormones have some influence over hunger, cravings, energy and mood.
Using the phrase "count up your hormones" is a good a way to grab your attention, and in this book, I am going to teach you exactly how to do this in the most efficient way.

When you start off with a hormonal approach to a fat loss diet, you soon will realize that the habit of eating becomes something that becomes a part of you. You know that it becomes a matter of eating more of the right things rather than less of anything else. Moreover, because everyone is different, the good things can vary from person to person.

Well perhaps you know somebody who eats large amounts of protein and fat, they then lost a ton of weight and were able to maintain that weight loss effortlessly. Perhaps you know somebody that have adopted an entirely vegetarian diet and were also able to achieve their perfect weight and they also maintained that body change.

They were successful because they stumbled across an approach that matched their metabolic expression, psychological sensitivities, and personal preferences. However, these people are in the minority. Most individuals in the real world are not so fortunate as the picture-perfect people on TV. We all have tried a bunch of weight loss programs, and we still can't find the solution to our problems. This is because many of us do not take a hormones-first approach to diet change but, we tend to take a calories-first approach rather than that.

The first step in a hormones-first approach is to begin eating a smarter calorie diet but not a lower calorie diet. My doctor told me that he had his patients start their treatment regimen by eating as much lean protein as they wish. They can have as many low-sugar fruits as they want (e.g., apples, pears, berries and bananas). The doctor told them they could have unlimited amounts of non-starchy vegetables. I then suggest limiting all starchy foods to no more than five to 15 bites at each of the three major meals such as breakfast, lunch and dinner, depending on what they could manage.

From there, the patients then learn to pay attention to how hungry they feel from each meal to meal. The would judge at what the strength and prevalence of their hunger cravings are. They then would rate by about how much energy they have. He had those people rank these sensations on a scale from 1-to-10, with 1 being low and 10 being high. The ideal state of hunger with a ratio (hunger and cravings) to both be less than five on the scale, and for energy to be 6 or better. It will compare the two on a scale.

I have heard it called a type of Metabolic Effect; some call this the HEC score (pronounced "hellish! HEC" That stands for Hunger, Energy, and Cravings). If any one of these biofeedback sensations does not meet this criterion, the detective work continues. You can have some Starches which may be changed up or down depending on your situation. Timing starches in the morning or for a post-workout may be determined to be good depending on your style. We then look at increasing, decreasing or eliminating the Fat and dairy foods depending on your hormone habits. You take a look at your Eating frequency and adjust accordingly. The end goal is to create a pattern that you can eat in a way that balances these HEC sensations that come up first. When you do, you know this way of eating can become a habit.

Once you find your HEC balance, then you focus on the fat. You can judge if you are losing fat in your body. You have reached success when you have found your fat-loss formula. If you are there yet, it is time to check again. You need to go over it again to adjust your diet accordingly. You need to Check your Meal frequency, your fat content, your starchy carbohydrates and some of the other dietary parameters are then adjusted to the inches you see begin to become less. Your ultimate goal is to get your HEC in balance and to achieve fat loss. This approach requires you being like a big detective, *not just* someone on a diet.
When HEC is in balance, and you are losing fat, you then can find a lifestyle for your body change. When this has become a habit, it will form a plan that you can be able to follow through with for a long time, rather than a quick diet, you may have tried before, just like a typical new year's resolution.

The next step is the dreaded Counting of the calories.

When I first had to do this in a physical science class, I was surprised by just how quickly the smallest meals added up to calories and how much exercise eliminated those calories. In the course, they gave an example of two women eating a little lunch at the mall and how many hours it would take for each woman based on height and weight to burn off those calories. They walked the mall for like 3 hours for an orange soda and one slice of pepperoni pizza.

People often find that the typical starving yourself diet to calories is not the best way to go. Let us start with you diet. You need a healthy diet for energy for daily activities. The human body needs many things from the items we eat such as iron, calcium, salt and more to maintain balance. It is not all about fat or no- fat. Most people find that they are naturally in a calorie deficit, which means they need more of a different type of calorie. Less they may find that they are consuming more calories on an average that they were before. This does not matter because they believe that they are in a balanced metabolic state, and they are losing weight. They think that calories do not matter.

To reiterate, by counting up your hormones rather than up your calories that means that you are now taking a hormones-first approach and not calories-first approach. Rather than indiscriminately cutting calories and dealing with the constant hunger, constant hunger cravings and low energy that come with it that approach. When you use your food to balance scale for these sensations, you are operating from a place of some strength. Moreover, you can do it and stick to the program.

Some Quick points.
1. Begin to change your way of eating, by eating more foods that suppress your hunger, control cravings and that gives you more energy. These foods do not have magic burn away fat particles in them they make you more energetic for you to be able to achieve fat loss from your caloric diet and the hormone balance.
2. Look at your HEC score. After you do that every day and then adjust your diet based on your needs and goals. You need to meet your hunger goal and cravings goal consistently below 5 and energy consistently above 6.
3. Start by Measuring your fat loss. This process is accomplished mainly by assessing how many inches you have lost, not by how many pounds that you have shed. If you find that your fat-loss is not what you want, adjust your eating approach to food. while you are maintaining your HEC score in the balanced zone. Be more like a weight loss detective, than someone just on a diet.
4. When you have achieved some fat loss and an HEC that is balanced, you have found what they call your metabolic effect on your body.

Bonus: This process helps you with the changes both reliably navigate and the inevitable metabolic changes of pregnancy, menopause, stress, and aging.

3. Chapter 2: The Metabolic Types

There is a Great Questionnaire that you can take on line at
https://www.totalgym.com/Images/Product/Documents/Life%20Survey_Spec.pdf

How to Determine Your Metabolic Body Type and you want To Feed It
    To begin, you must learn how to determine your metabolic body type. We all have different metabolic types, and you may also have a particular kind of body metabolism that affects your body type, line, and personality. If you eat according to your metabolic type, you will feel better, look better, and you will live a healthier lifestyle.

How to determine your metabolic type?

Why some studies that claim that foods used beyond, inside or

    One nutrition plan that was determined to prove in a study where certain food that were used as medicine in the body, Clearly, not every food that you eat works for every body type of metabolism. Many studies show that when you are born, you possess a particular kind of blood group, a particular form of the body. There is also a particular type of metabolism for you too. This explains why person a can eat some food and then feels healthy and looks great, but person b, can eat the same foods and then see weight gain and fatigue. Have you ever had a friend that seem to eat like a horse and still be hungry and you look at food and have to adjust your belt?

Here is how to measure your metabolic type using these three basic types of metabolism – A, B, and C.

A good healthy diet should have plenty of fresh fruits and vegetables, Carbohydrates, fat, and proteins.

The type A – Metabolism

If like salty foods such as potato chips and are prone to anxiety, then you more than likely did not notice that this constant feeling of anxiety was because of the salty and fatty foods that you are eating.

Here are some of the most common characteristics of a person with body type A metabolism:

- Having an appetite, that is strong.
- A continued craving for fatty and salty snack foods
- Having anxiety and fatigue
- openness towards people and verbosity

So How should a person with Type-A Metabolic body type eat food and how much of each type of foods?
  That is a really good Question to answer.
    A person with the Type-A Metabolic body type eats food and how much of each type of foods should be about half of protein about thirty percent of fat and about twenty percent of carbohydrates
This Type-A Metabolic person burns fat and proteins much easier than they consume carbohydrates. The hunger cravings for the salty and fatty foods comes from the body's needs for protein.

A good meal again should be 20% carbohydrates, 30% fats, and 50% proteins.

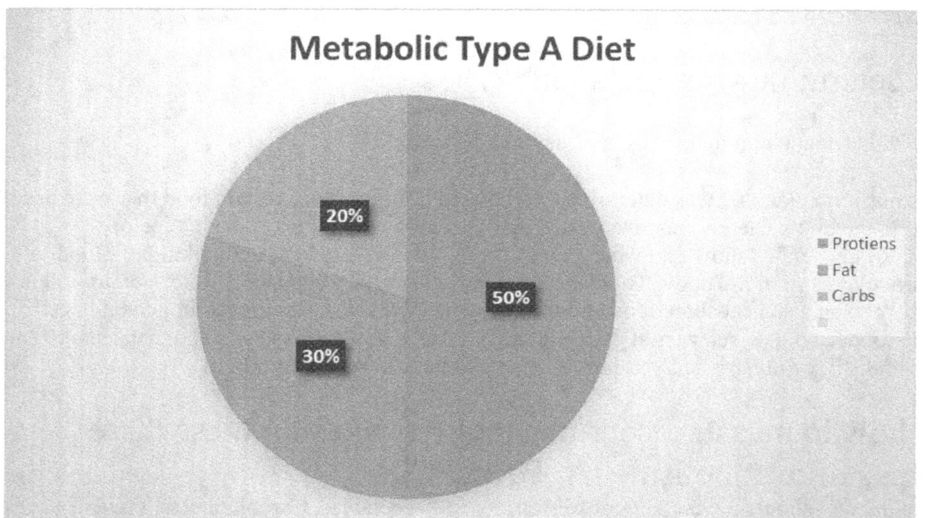

Turkey, Chicken, are some lean proteins with darker colors. It is good to eat Fish, such as tuna or salmon, can be an excellent choice and even occasionally consume some beef too.
The Type- A metabolic body type person should drink milk with 2% fat milk, whole milk, and eggs. These foods are a better choice for you than low-fat ones that are full of additional sugar.
Remember that you need a full-fat dairy product in your diet and they are a much healthier that eating salty and greasy snacks.
If you want to satisfy your metabolism, then you need to acknowledge what your body needs. In your case, it is a necessity of fat in the body. Eat various fresh fruits and veggies, but avoid eating processed foods which are full of sugar and may increase your anxiety. You can switch potatoes and white bread for whole grain bread and pasta.

The type B – Metabolism

If you are the type B metabolism, then you crave for sweets instead such as cakes, ice cream, cake, and cookies. Your body needs healthy carbohydrates, but your passion is currently focused on refined sugar most.

Essential characteristics of a person with type B metabolism are

They may have Poor appetite

Usually has a Craving for some sweets

A variety of sensitivity

They have high stress levels

Many times, they are dependent on caffeine

Many times, these people have difficulty with weight loss

A good meal again should be 70% carbohydrates, 10% fats, and 20% proteins. Type-B Metabolic person should eat low fat and low- protein diet. This diet should have healthy carbohydrates, whole grains with fresh fruits, and vegetables.

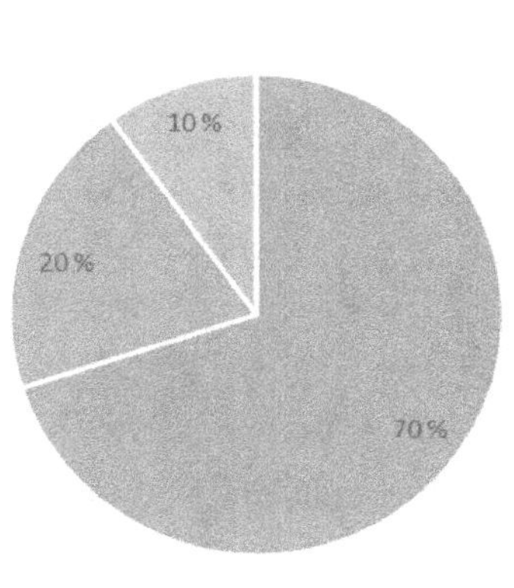

Most people would like to have their diet based on carbohydrates.

The whole grains should give you a certain amount of protein. You should keep that in mind, so you do not want to neglect them entirely. You can eat brown rice, whole grain bread, barley, pasta from whole grains and things like that. You can eat chicken, turkey, plants that are rich in proteins, such as chickpeas and lentils, and white fish. You should eat low fat dairy products. To help with the reducing the dependence of caffeine, you can switch to green tea, which also has a small portion of caffeine in it but is a healthier and wiser comparative to drinking a cup of Joe.

The type C – Metabolism

By now If you have not found your type in any of the previous models, such as you having a craving for sweet and savory alike, then it more likely you are in the C-type metabolism.

The C- Type of metabolism is a combination of both metabolic type A and B, and it includes the following features:
You have an unpredictable and variable appetite.
You may have cravings for sweet and savory or spicy
You may have Fatigue and Anxiety
Some have a little trouble maintaining their weight.

The C-Type metabolism person's diet should be a good balance of Proteins, Fats, and Carbohydrates equally. They usually have a good combustion of all three; that is why there is a craving for Savory and sweet.

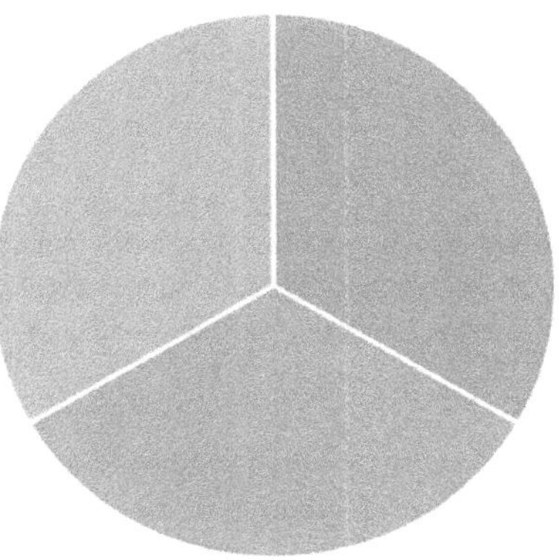

Equally Thirty-Three percent of Carbohydrates, Fats, and Proteins.

The C- Type Metabolic person can consume most types of fats.

They can have a combination of Low-fat and whole milk products, such as yogurt, low fat cheese, olive oil, and more. They can eat chicken, beef, turkey, salmon, soy and beans.

They should look for carbohydrates in the store where to get whole grains and certain types of Veggies and fruits, such as bananas or sweet potatoes.

Some foods help to speed up Your Metabolism!

Here is a list of some great foods to help you do, just that!

Some foods actually help with burning calories. While the food is in the digestion processing of the body, there are some of the foods that the body needs to use more energy to process. Those foods then burn more calories to do so, which stores less fat in the body.

Some foods make you reduce the risk of weight gain during the winter months.

Following is a list formula from page one of the Natural Health Yellow Pages. Hopefully, this can help you determine your type and what you can best use depending on you.

1. **Yogurt**. - This is rich in calcium which can increase the metabolism speed rate. If you do not have enough calcium in your body, it will increasingly store calories and fat. Yogurt has fifty percent more calcium than milk. It also helps to strengthen your immune system. Yogurt is a pro biotic which can reduce the risk of the accumulation of fat in the abdomen. Your daily consumption of yogurt should be three minimal.

2. **Salmon**. – Fish such as salmon have omega-3 fatty acids that can help you to build muscle and the more muscle you have, the more of the burning of the calories; you will find. Omega 3 fatty acids may reduce cortisol in the body that is a stress hormone. The Stress hormones let people say it is o.k. to nibble and overeat. The weekly recommendation of oily fish is 85 grams.

3. **Beans**. - Excellent source of resistant starch and fiber. This helps the body to burn off more calories. Many scientists have discovered that food that contains resistant starch such as **beans, bananas, and lentils** can increase burning calories by up to 24%. You should eat one or two servings a day of foods like that.

4. **Avocado**. - Avocados are excellent because they contain antioxidants and unsaturated fatty acids as well as 14 grams of fiber that encourage calorie burning. This can keep the rate of metabolism to a fast pace. The body should be protecting itself from infection and maintaining the cardiovascular system. You can have at least two times a day food that have healthy fats like the avocado.

5. **Hot Peppers**- That hot feeling that comes from capsaicin, which can stimulate the body to burn calories 50-100 times, right after eating them. You can eat hot chilies for your needs. If they are too hot, then you do not need to overeat them. Chile peppers also have some vitamin C in them.

6. **Coffee**. -Can be helpful in the morning when you wake up. The Coffee will speed up your metabolism and stimulates the nervous system and promotes burning calories. It is hard to determine how much coffee is recommended. It depends on how the caffeine affects you.

7. **Green Tea**. -Has a compound called EGCG and it Contains antioxidant catechin and caffeine. This stimulates the nervous system and promotes burning calories. Many studies shown that drinking green tea helps weight loss. Like coffee, it is hard to determine how much coffee is recommended. It depends on how the caffeine affects you.

8. **Egg whites** -Egg whites are rich in branched-chain amino acids. Amino Acids, which keep your metabolism stoked, says Chicago nutritionist David Grotto, RDN. Eggs are full of Vitamin D and protein.

You only need to determine your metabolic diet and your type. Then you can learn how to better you're eating habits and speed up your system. Keep up the good work!

4. Chapter 3: Some Recipes

Banana Nut Job Breakfast Smoothies

Here is a quick breakfast for people on the go that is jam packed with healthy fats, proteins and potassium to get you up and moving toward a great day!

Ingredients

7 oz. 2% plain Greek **Yogurt**
1 tbsp. of almond butter
½ **banana**
1 tbsp. flaxseed oil or ground flaxseed
Ice to help make the smoothie thick

Directions

1. Put items in blender

2. Blend ingredients until smooth

3. Many people like to add additional toppings (some suggestions are, ½ cup blueberries with two teaspoons of ginger, 1 cup of chopped kale with ½ teaspoon of turmeric, or ½ cup of strawberries/ raspberries with one teaspoon with some vanilla extract.

The Sweetest Honey Garlic Lemon Salmon

1 1/2 pounds' fillets of **salmon**
 You need lemon pepper and Garlic powder to add a salty flavor
1/3 cup soy sauce
1/3 cup brown sugar
 1/3 cup water
You can add **chicken** flavoring to give it an added boost.
1/4 cup vegetable oil Add all ingredients to list
A few Drops of natural honey
A dash of Lemon and Herb Seasoning

Prep time, approx. 15 minutes
Cook time 16 minutes
Ready in about 2 hours and a half
First, you need to season the fillets of salmon with the lemon pepper, garlic powder, and the salt.

Then in a small bowl, you stir together soy sauce, brown sugar, water, and vegetable oil and a few drops of honey until sugar is dissolved into the seasoning solution. Then place each fillet of fish into a large resealable plastic bag with the sauce mixture. Seal the fillets and then turn them over to coat.

Then put them in the refrigerator for about 2 hours.

Preheats your grill to heat that is about medium.

Then lightly oil the grill and place the salmon on the preheated grill. You can discard the marinade.

Cook the Salmon for approx. 6 minutes to 8 minutes per side, or until the fish is flaky and easy to get with a fork.

Many people use Aluminum foil to keep food moist, cook it evenly, and make clean-up easier.

The Meanie Greenie salad
Ingredients
Two tablespoons olive oil
Two tablespoons fresh lime juice
Two tablespoons mango chutney
One tablespoon low-sodium soy sauce
3/4 teaspoon grated peeled fresh ginger
4 (4-ounce) skinless, boneless chicken-breast halves
Cooking spray
8 cups mixed salad **greens**
1 cup diced peeled **mango**
3/4 cup diced peeled **avocado**

Basic directions
1. Prepare grill.
2. Combine oil, juice, chutney, soy sauce, and ginger in a small bowl.
Place chicken on large plate; spoon two tablespoons oil mixture over chicken, reserving the rest for the salad.
Turn chicken to coat, and let stand 5 minutes.
3. Place chicken on grill rack coated with cooking spray;
grill 4 minutes on each side or until chicken is done, brushing with oil mixture from the plate before turning the chicken.
 Slice chicken crosswise into strips.
4. Arrange greens, mango, and **avocado** on four serving plates.
 Arrange chicken over greens.
Drizzle reserved dressing over salads.

The Ultimate Bean and rice!

1 cup uncooked white rice
2 cups water
1 Tbsp. Olive oil
1/2 cup chopped red bell pepper
1/2 cup chopped green pepper
1/2 cup chopped sweet onion
One clove garlic minced fine
3/4 cup tomato sauce
Two tsp ground cumin
1/2 tsp dried oregano
1/4 tsp salt
Two 15-oz cans black beans, rinsed and drained
2 Tbsp. vinegar
This is a quick lunch meal.
Prep Time: 10 minutes
Cook Time: 20 minutes
Total Time: 30 minutes

Step one.
To prepare the rice, combine the rice and the water in a large saucepan over high heat.
Bring the water to a boil.
Put the heat on medium and simmer for twenty minutes, or until the rice is tender.

While the rice is cooking, proceed with making the **beans**
Step Two.

Pour the olive oil into a large heavy skillet,
The heat in the skillet should be turned to medium-high heat.
Add to the skillet, the chopped red bell pepper, chopped green bell pepper, chopped onion, and minced garlic.

Continue cooking the vegetables for 8 minutes, or until the vegetables are tender.
 Then, add the tomato sauce, the ground cumin, the oregano, and the salt.
Turn the heat to medium, and simmer the mixture for 5 minutes. Then, add the black beans and the vinegar, and simmer an additional 10 minutes.
Step Three
. To serve, spoon about 1/3 cup of cooked rice into each bowl, and then ladle the beans equally into each bowl, on top of the rice.

This dish should Serves 6 people

Per Serving Calories 259, Fat 3 grams, Pro 10 grams, Carbs 48 grams

5. Chapter 4: Healthy Warnings! What to Not Eat or Drink

I was researching foods to avoid, and I found that Doctor Karen Shackleford has a great story about her weight with her lifelong diet of gains and losses, that with mostly weight gains, which she stated had reached her height at 205 pounds. After she and her family had been on a juicing diet for a few weeks, they all felt hungry and miserable. She stated that she found herself passing by a fast food place and thinking if she just chewed on some fries and spat them out that, then it would not count as intake calories. Then she stated that the best tasting meal of her life with fries, a strawberry shake, and a thick double bacon cheeseburger ended her juicing diet.

Later she was at her work having lunch with a coworker when she was just sipping on a diet soda and the co-worker stated to her with a plate full of food. Her colleague said that she loved food, but just ate the right kinds of food, in the right amounts at the right time of day. The co-worker did not believe in dieting. She just talked about what to eat and when.

Some items to Just Plain Avoid all together according to Doctor Karen Shackleford
1. Orange Juice- She stated that it shocked her to hear this too. We all have heard to start your day with O.J. She says that concentrated orange juice is one of the most harmful things that you can eat or drink. Most Concentrated Fruit Juices, like cranberries, apple, and grape can cause problems around the waistline.

   Explanation: Doctor Shackleford Stated that this cannot be right. Did she ask herself? Isn't fruit healthy? This cannot be. After she had conducted some research, she found that it is not the fruit but the process the companies use to concentrate the juice.

   The Companies remove the fiber and other nutrients out of fruit during the "concentrating process." The fiber in fruit typically reduces the spike in blood sugar. With the fiber is taken out then, we are primarily left with sugar water.

   When your blood sugar is too high, it puts your body into fat storing mode.

   This method just basically tells your body that anything you eat needs to be stored as fat.

   Your blood sugar levels are related to your insulin levels. Insulin is also known as your fat storing Hormone. Most concentrated juices have as much and sometimes even more sugar than soda. Many processed foods have excess amounts of sugar in them.

   Some names of this excess sugar you may have seen on labels

   - High Fructose Corn Syrup
   - Dextran
   - Dextrose
   - Fruit Juice Concentrate

2. Margarine – It has trans fats which usually have hydrogen added to them, so they do not spoil. Eating these trans fats can increase the risk of cardiovascular disease as well as weight gain. Trans fats also increase your LDL or Bad Cholesterol. Sometimes wiping out your HDL or Good Cholesterol, by building up plaque in your arteries. A Good alternative to Margarine is Butter.

   Butter has fat in it as well. The fat in butter is a saturated fat that your body can burn up as fuel instead of building plaque in your arteries like trans fats do.

3. Whole wheat bread- Doctor stated that this is a shock to her as well. Not just whole wheat bread but other bread in the carbohydrates categories, that High Carbohydrate "comfort foods" that we love such as apple pie, cakes, muffins, pasta, and pizza.

   You do not have to give up the foods that you love.

   She stated that she gave up sweets and began to exercise. She said that she lost some weight but could not get rid of the belly. Many times, life would just get too busy for some of that.

   There is an old saying that "you cannot exercise your way out of poor nutrition."

   That means that no amount of exercise can help you if you are not eating nutrient dense foods that your body needs to metabolize.

   When Carbohydrates combine with other foods in the body like proteins, it does not raise your blood sugar level and does not put your body into fat storing mode.
   She stated that her family might have a typical meal that might be a stack of syrup pancakes for breakfast, a cheeseburger for lunch and fried or broiled chicken with rice for dinner. Before she found out how to eat. In her example, she had a plate full of High carbs for breakfast. Which again raising her sugar levels that just tells her body to store everything you eat as fat.

   She then tells that it is not The High-Carbs that was the problem but the amount and lack of other things. So, then she just had to customize her meals to add the right balance of proteins, with some low carbs, and the high carbs, to balance the meals and keep her sugar level.

   She stated that when she did this. She could still have that burger for lunch and her chicken dinner. When many people diet they do not eat enough and then their body is in fat storing mode because it thinks that you are starving. To preserve your life, anything that you eat will go into fat storing mode. So, you need balance to burn off the weight. Starving yourself will not help. Because when you do eat you, the body will store it as fat.

   As you, gain weight, your body tends to produce less, adiponectin which is your body's natural fat burner. Then add in your day to day stress which we all live with, and the excess cortisol your body produces because of the stress and you can see why weight loss can be so difficult.

   Green tea has been proven to increase levels of adiponectin, aside from its fat burning powers, Green Tea is a natural anti-inflammatory, which can sometimes help ease swelling with weight gain.

4. Ghrelin is like the lazy lion that is ready to pounce. It is the compound in your body that lets you raid the refrigerator 1 hour after eating a fast food meal like a hungry lion. One way to reduce the Ghrelin in the body is to eat certain nutrient-dense foods instead of processed soy products. Like cinnamon and blueberries.
Ghrelin

Ghrelin is produced by the stomach. Among its numerous functions, ghrelin increases appetite and stimulates the release of growth hormone.
What is ghrelin?
Ghrelin is a hormone that is produced and released mainly by the stomach with small amounts also released by the small intestine, pancreas and brain.

Ghrelin has numerous functions. It is termed the 'hunger hormone' because it stimulates appetite, increases food intake and promotes fat storage. When administered to humans, ghrelin increases food intake by up to 30% by circulating in the bloodstream at the hypothalamus, an area of the brain crucial in the control of appetite. Recently, ghrelin has also been shown to act on regions of the brain involved in reward processing such as the amygdala.

Ghrelin also stimulates the release of growth hormone from the pituitary gland, which, unlike ghrelin itself, breaks down fat tissue and causes the build-up of muscle.

Ghrelin also has protective effects on the cardiovascular system and plays a role in the control of insulin release.

How is ghrelin controlled?
Ghrelin levels are primarily regulated by food intake. Levels of ghrelin in the blood rise just before eating and when fasting, with the timing of these rises being affected by our normal meal routine. Hence, ghrelin is thought to play a role in mealtime 'hunger pangs' and the need to begin meals. Levels of ghrelin increase when fasting (in line with increased hunger) and are lower in individuals with a higher body weight compared with lean individuals, which suggests ghrelin could be involved in the long-term regulation of body weight.

Eating reduces concentrations of ghrelin. Different nutrients slow down ghrelin release to varying degrees; carbohydrates and proteins restrict the production and release of ghrelin to a greater extent than fats.
Somatostatin also restricts ghrelin release, as well as many other hormones released from the digestive tract.
What happens if I have too much ghrelin?
Ghrelin levels increase after dieting, which may explain why diet-induced weight loss can be difficult to maintain. One would expect higher levels in people with obesity. However, ghrelin levels are usually lower in people with higher body weight compared with lean people, which suggests ghrelin is not a cause of obesity; although there is a suggestion that obese people are actually more sensitive to the hormone. However, more research is needed to confirm this.

Prader-Willi syndrome is a genetic disease in which patients have severe obesity, extreme hunger and learning difficulties. Unlike more common forms of obesity, circulating ghrelin levels are high in

Prader-Willi syndrome patients and start before the development of obesity. This suggests that ghrelin may contribute to their increased appetite and body weight.

Ghrelin levels are also high in cachexia and the eating disorder, anorexia nervosa. This may be the body's way of making up for weight loss by stimulating food intake and fat storage.

What happens if I have too little ghrelin?
Gastric bypass surgery, which involves reducing the size of the stomach, is considered to be the most effective treatment for severe, life-threatening obesity. Patients who lose weight after bypass surgery have been found to have lower ghrelin levels than those who lose weight by other means such as diet and exercise, which may partly explain the long-lasting success of this treatment.

5. Avoid GM Corn. This is not the regular run of the mill corn. It is banned in many countries. It is used to fatten up livestock so it is not a surprise that it does the same to us. Just one sweetener made from GM corn makes a big contribution to the obesity and diabetes epidemic. This harmful sweetener is hiding in many places that you would never expect it.

Such as in

Breads and cereals
Cottage cheese and yogurt
Salad dressings
Drinks made with organic fruit juice
Fast food sandwiches

It is no surprise that food that sits on a self has things in it to make it last longer. Processed foods are not the answer.

6. Conclusion:

We hope that you find a diet buddy, a forum or a community, a trainer, or a friend to help you stay on track. We all know how difficult it can be to diet alone. We don't want you to give up everything that you love. Just to find the right combination of foods, at the right times with the right amounts and you will be more than surprised by your results.

Thank you and we Wish you all well.

T.W. Flora

7. Research References:

Various references to the metabolic diet from the internet pieced together.
Day-Off Diet Almond Butter Banana Smoothie.
 (n.d.). Retrieved from http://top.adlesse.com/en/i/593830606284272444/day-off-diet-almond-butter-banana
Crispy beans and rice ten-minute chicken tacos from. recipe.
 (n.d.). Retrieved from http://recipes100.com/recipe+crispy+beans+and+rice+ten+minute+chicken+tacos+from
Grilled Chicken Salad with Avocado and Mango Recipe
 (n.d.). Retrieved from http://www.myrecipes.com/recipe/grilled-chicken-salad-with-avocado-mango

Other Good references:
Peer-reviewed research references
1) - Jason Gill and Naveed Sattar; "Fruit Juice: just another sugary drink?" The Lancet Diabetes & Endocrinology, online 10 February 2014; DOI:10.1016/S2213-8587(14)70013-0.
2) - Hermansen, K and Mortensen LS, "Bodyweight changes associated with antihyperglycemic agents in type 2 diabetes mellitus", Drug Safety, 2007;30(12):1127-42.
- Khan, Rehman and Russell-Jones, David, "Insulin-associated weight-gain in diabetes, causes, effects, and coping strategies," Diabetes, Obesity, and Metabolism, 2007; DOI: 10.1111/j.1463-1326.2006.00686.x
3) - Food and Drug Administration, "Guidance for Industry: Action Levels for Poisonous or Deleterious Substances in Human Food and
Animal Feed", FDA Website, August 2000.
4) - Murphy SL, Xu JQ, Kochanek KD. Deaths: Final data for 2010. Natl Vital Stat Rep. 2013;61(4).
- Go AS, Mozaffarian D, Roger VL, Benjamin EJ, Berry JD, Blaha MJ, et al. Heart disease and stroke statistics—2014 update:
a report from the American Heart Association. Circulation. 2014;128.
- Heidenreich PA, Trogdon JG, Khavjou OA, et al. Forecasting the future of cardiovascular disease in the United States: a policy statement from the American Heart Association. Circulation. 2011; 123:933-44. Epub 2011 Jan 24.